All rights reserved. No part of this publication maybe reproduced, distributed, or transmitted in any formor by any means, including photocopying, recording, or other electronic or mechanical methods, without the prior written permission of the publisher, except in the case of brief quotations embodied in critical reviews and certain other noncommercial uses permitted by copyright law.

Contents

What are oxalates? 6

What does our body do to the oxalates? 6

What is a low oxalate diet? 7

Which are low oxalate foods? 8

What are the benefits of a low oxalic diet? 9

Tips to follow a low oxalic diet 12

What foods should I limit or avoid? 14

What other dietary guidelines should I follow?. 17

Kitchen Chicken Piccata 18

Granola 20

Vegetable Casserole 22

Southwestern Quinoa 25

Chicken Mulligatawny Soup 27

Classic English Toad-in-the-Hole................... 32

Portuguese Salt Cod Stew (Bacalao or Bacalhoada).. 35

Brazilian Salmon Stew (Moqueca).................. 41

Moqueca – Brazilian Fish Stew 45

Rabbit Braised in Belgian Ale........................ 61

Winter Chicken Salad with Tangy Miso Dressing 67

Teriyaki Chicken Breasts 71

Miso Glazed Salmon..................................... 75

Easy Weeknight Chicken Ramen 78

Pan Simmered Pacific Black Cod 83

Tempura Fried Calamari 86

Seared Ahi Tuna.. 91

Ambrosia Salad 94

Apple and Sweet Potato Matzo Bake 97

Charoset with Apples, Dates, and Walnuts 101

Apple Galette with Blue Cheese, Almonds and Honey 103

Gruyere, Apple, and Fig Jam Panini.............. 109

Vegan Sweet Potatoes................................ 111

Thai Chicken 113

Grilled Halibut with Fennel Sauce Recipe 115

Truffle Custard with Crab and Caviar Recipe . 120

Tomato-Basil Crab Bisque Recipe................. 124

Stuffed Snow Peas with Crab Recipe 128

She Crab Soup History and Recipe............... 130

Taverna Opa's Steamed King Crab Legs Recipe 137

Hot Artichoke and Crab Appetizer Recipe 141

Gourmet Hot Crab Dip Recipe 143

Basil & lemon chickpeas with mackerel 146

Easy Tomato Soup 149

PASTA SALAD WITH BAKED TINGA SALMON . 152

What are oxalates?

Oxalates are also known as oxalic acid, is a chemical compound naturally found in our body. They are present in a variety of plant foods like green leafy vegetables, fruits, nuts, and seeds. They are present in low quantities in dairy food, meat, and poultry food.

What does our body do to the oxalates?

Oxalates are not so essential for our body, so it binds to the other waste products in food and makes their way to the kidneys to excrete it out. Oxalates often bind to minerals such as calcium and are excreted out of the body through urine and stool.

However, when we consume excessive oxalates, our body fails to flush it through urine, especially if you are not drinking enough fluids. As oxalates increases in the body, they can bind to calcium and block the absorption of minerals, form crystals and eventually kidney stone.

Hence to avoid these consequences, your doctor often advice you to have a low oxalate diet. But what does it mean?

What is a low oxalate diet?

A low oxalate diet refers to a diet from which the amount of oxalate does not exceed 50 grams per day. If you plan your diet properly, then you can do it. In addition to limiting your oxalate intake, staying well-hydrated, moderating your protein intake, and increasing calcium consumption are other essential aspects of a low-oxalate diet. Typically, doctors recommended, to follow the diet for at least 3-6 weeks to see if your symptoms improve.

Which are low oxalate foods?

There are plenty of low oxalate foods that are available easily and can enjoy as a part of a healthy diet. Here are some top low oxalate food that you can add to your diet –

- Dairy products – Milk, cheese, yogurt, butter, and buttermilk

- Fruits – avocado, banana, cherries, mango, papaya, passion fruit, grapes, and melons

- Vegetables – cauliflower, cabbages, radish, mushrooms, cucumber, and peas

- Grains – white rice, barley, oat bran, and corn bran

- Herbs and spices – rosemary, basil, turmeric, cumin, and ginger

- Beverages – water, herbal tea, apple cider vinegar, and wine

- Poultry food – eggs and chicken

- Meat products (Avoid processed meat)

What are the benefits of a low oxalic diet?

1: Prevent the formation of kidney stones.

When oxalate concentration increase in your body, calcium oxalate stone will develop in your kidney. Various research suggests that almost 75% of kidney stones developed from calcium oxalate. A better pathway to excrete oxalate is from the stool as it will not bind to calcium and prevent the formation of kidney stones.

2: Reduce the risk of cystic fibrosis complication

Cystic fibrosis (CF) is a hereditary lung and digestive disorder where the body produces thick and sticky mucus that can clog the lungs and obstruct the pancreas. Though cystic fibrosis is untreatable and unavoidable, we can lower the risk of complications.

In cystic fibrosis patients, doctors always recommend consuming low oxalate foods because to avoid further complications named- hyperoxaluria. The research found that 51% of cystic fibrosis patients had hyperoxaluria, and this is a dangerous risk factor for kidney stones.

3: Prevent underactive thyroid problems

When the body contains excess oxalate, it will store in various tissues and thyroid. This excess oxalate binds to a hormone released from the thyroid – T3 leads to formations of crystals in the thyroid. This crystal reduces the activity of the thyroid gland, leads to the development of various symptoms such as weight gain, fatigue, high cholesterol level, menstrual problems, etc. Hence, it always better to consume oxalate-containing food within a limit.

4: Helpful for autism patients

Researchers have suggested that individuals with autism may be predisposed to oxalate intolerance. Although the metabolic pathways are unclear, individuals with autistic tendencies have seen an improvement in their symptoms when consuming a low oxalate diet.

Tips to follow a low oxalic diet

1: Moderate consumption of high-oxalate diet

Minimizing high-oxalate food from your diet could potentially help to prevent kidney stones. Research suggests that increasing your intake of calcium could boost oxalate excretion and may be more effective against kidney stones. Here are some sample oxalate-calcium combos to try-

- Berries with yogurt

- Broccoli with feta cheese

- Quinoa and chia seeds with milk (to make overnight breakfast quinoa)

2: Enjoy low oxalate foods

Various low oxalate foods help to lower your oxalate levels to enjoy it. In a low oxalate diet, you can include avocado, cauliflower, herbal tea, dairy products, chicken, and meat.

3: Consume calcium-rich foods

Oxalate and calcium bind together to prevent the formation of kidney stones. Therefore it's recommended to pair your oxalate diet with high-calcium-containing foods like yogurt and cheese.

4: Drink plenty of water

Water helps to flush many toxic substances from your body through your kidney and helps to prevent the formation of kidney stones. It is advisable to drink at least eight 8-ounce glasses of water or fluids per day.

5: Avoid excessive sodium in diet

Sodium causes the body to hold on to water, which counteracts the oxalate-flushing benefits of healthy hydration.

6: Cut down excess vitamin C supplementation

When you consume vitamin C, it breaks down into your body and forms oxalates. If you are taking an excessive amount of vitamin C, then oxalate may get accumulated in your body and will produce various health issues.

What foods should I limit or avoid?

Limit the following foods that are high in oxalate.

- Grains:

o Wheat bran, wheat germ, and barley

o Grits and bran cereal

- White corn flour and buckwheat flour
  - Whole wheat bread
- Fruit:
  - Dried apricots
  - Red currants, figs, and rhubarb
  - Kiwi
- Vegetables:
  - Collard greens, leeks, okra, and spinach
  - Wax beans
  - Eggplant
  - Beets and beet greens
  - Swiss chard, escarole, parsley, and rutabagas
  - Tomato paste

- Protein foods:

  o Baked beans with tomato sauce

  o Nut butters and nuts (peanuts, almonds, pecans, cashews, hazelnuts)

  o Soy burgers

  o Miso

  o Dried beans

- Desserts:

  o Fruitcake

  o Chocolate

  o Carob and marmalade

- Beverages:

  o Chocolate drink mixes

- Soy milk
  - Instant iced tea
- Other foods:
  - Sesame seeds and tahini (paste made of sesame seeds)
  - Poppy seeds

What other dietary guidelines should I follow?

- Drink about 12 to 16 (eight-ounce) cups of liquid each day. Liquids help clear kidney stones and prevent them from forming again. Water is the best liquid to drink. You may need more liquid if you are physically active. Ask your healthcare provider or dietitian how much liquid you need to drink each day.

- Your healthcare provider may suggest that you make other diet changes to help prevent kidney stones. This may include decreasing the amount of sodium you eat each day.

Kitchen Chicken Piccata

INGREDIENTS

- 2 chicken breasts, pounded thin or butterflied
- 1/4 cup water chestnut flour
- 6 Tbsp butter
- 4 Tbsp olive oil
- 1/2 cup chicken stock
- 1/4 cup fresh lemon juice
- 3 Tbsp capers, rinsed

- 2 Tbsp fresh parsley, chopped

- 2 cloves garlic, chopped

Instructions

1. Add olive oil and 4 tbsp of the butter to a saute pan on medium to high heat. Dredge the chicken cutlets in the flour and, when the butter is melted, add to the pan. Cook for a few minutes on each side, until the chicken is lightly browned on the outside and cooked through in the middle.

2. Set the chicken aside, put the other 2 tbsp butter in the pan, and add the garlic. Let it cook for about a minute, being careful not to let it burn. Add the chicken stock, lemon juice and capers, and let the mixture cook for a few more minutes.

3. Add the chicken back into the sauce, just long enough for the chicken to reheat. Garnish with fresh parsley and enjoy!

Granola

INGREDIENTS

- 1.25 teaspoon vanilla extract

- 2 tablespoons vegetable oil

- 3 cups rolled old fashioned oats gluten-free if gluten intolerant

- 1.5 teaspoon ground cinnamon

- 1/2 cup unsalted sunflower seeds

- 1/2 cup unsalted pistachios

- 1/4 teaspoon kosher salt

- 2 Tablespoons sugar-free pancake syrup

- 1/2 Cup no sugar added dried cranberries

INSTRUCTIONS

1. Preheat oven to 325 degrees.

2. In a large bowl, combine oats, sunflower seeds, dried cranberries, pistachios, oil, pancake syrup, and vanilla extract. Stir together with a spatula until evenly mixed.

3. Add in the cinnamon and salt, mix together.

4. Line a baking sheet with parchment paper and lightly spray with cooking spray.

5. Pour granola onto the baking sheet, making sure it's evenly distributed.

6. Bake for 10 minutes, then stir, bake another 5 minutes, until golden brown.

7. Remove and let cool.

Vegetable Casserole

Ingredients

- Squash sauce (recipe), homemade or store bought

- Sliced zucchini or squash, (one of each) or (minimum one medium zucchini)

- One bag of frozen Cauliflower florets

- 1/2 cup Grated Parmesan cheese (use more if you are a cheese fan)

- 1 small chopped onion

- 1 small chopped pepper (1/2 cup moderate oxalate))

- Crushed saltines (one sleeve) or breadcrumbs

- Salt and or white pepper to taste

INSTRUCTIONS

1. I use either a smaller rectangle 7 X 11 " glass baking dish or an eight inch square glass dish.

2. A 13 X 9 baking dish can be used to serve a larger crowd, but the ingredients need to be increased by 25 percent(ish.) This is a very flexible dish and can be tweaked with quantity or vegetable; all work!

3. Coat the glass dish with cooking spray.

4. Add one layer of sliced zucchini or sliced zucchini and squash

5. Add the onions and peppers and cauliflower florets on top of the zucchini layer.

6. Pour the squash sauce over the vegetables, sprinkle with parmesan and crushed saltines.

7. Cheese alert! I am very generous with the cheese and liberally sprinkle the cheese on each layer so I use 1/2 cup in total. A 1/4 cup of cheese after the zucchini layer and then on top of all the vegetables before the crunchy topping is added.

8. The layered vegetable casserole is now ready for the oven.

9. Bake at 350 degrees for approximately 50 minutes. Zucchini and squash bake quicker than the cauliflower so check the dish for doneness by inserting a fork into the vegetables. The vegetables should be fork tender.

10. If additional cooking time is necessary, I cover the dish with foil as I do not want the

crunchy saltine top to over brown. I baked the dish another 20 minutes.

11. Give the vegetables another fork test for tenderness. I prefer softer vegetables, but if a firmer vegetable is preferred then baking for 50 minutes total works well.

Southwestern Quinoa

Ingredients

- 1 cup quinoa rinsed

- 15 oz low sodium canned black beans drained & rinsed

- 2 plum tomatoes chopped

- 1 cup frozen corn thawed

- 1 red bell pepper chopped

- 2 green onions chopped
- 1/2 small red onion chopped
- 1/2 cup fresh cilantro chopped
- 1 lime juiced
- 1/3 cup olive oil
- 1/2 tsp salt
- 1/4 tsp black pepper
- 1 tsp chili powder
- 3 tbsp honey
- 3 tbsp white vinegar

Instructions

1. Cook quinoa according to package instructions. Do not add salt! There will be plenty of flavor from the dressing and veggies!

2. While quinoa is cooking, combine beans, tomatoes, corn, green onions, red bell pepper, red onion and cilantro in a large bowl.

3. Make dressing by whisking together lime juice, olive oil, salt, pepper, chili powder, honey and vinegar.

4. Add cooked quinoa to bowl with veggies. Fold in dressing. Serve garnished with more fresh cilantro if desired. This quinoa is delicious served immediately, or cold.

Chicken Mulligatawny Soup

INGREDIENTS

- 2 tablespoons butter

- 1 tablespoon extra virgin olive oil

- 1 large onion, chopped (about 2 cups)

- 2 ribs celery, chopped (about 1 cup)
- 2 carrots, chopped (about 1 cup)
- 2 bay leaves
- 4 teaspoon yellow curry powder
- 1 1/4 pound (570 g) boneless, skinless chicken thighs, trimmed of visible fat
- 2 cups (475 ml) chicken stock
- 2 cups (475 ml) water
- 1 1/2 teaspoons kosher salt (or 1 teaspoon sea salt)
- 1/4 cup uncooked basmati rice
- 2 tart apples, cored, peeled, and chopped (about 2 cups)
- 1/4 (60 ml) cup heavy whipping cream

- 1/4 cup (60 ml) plain yogurt for garnish

- 1 tablespoon minced chives for garnish

METHODHIDE PHOTOS

1 Sauté onions, celery, carrots in olive oil and butter, add bay leaves, curry powder: Heat butter and olive oil on medium high heat in a large (4 to 5 quart), thick-bottomed pot. Add the onions, celery, and carrots. Cook for 5 minutes until just starting to soften. Add the bay leaves. Add the curry powder and mix to coat.

2 Add chicken, stock, salt: Add the chicken thighs and stir to coat with the curry mixture. Add the stock and water to the pot. Add the salt. Bring to a simmer and reduce the heat to maintain a simmer. Cover and cook for 20 minutes.

3 Remove chicken, let cool to touch: Remove the chicken pieces from the pot. (They should be just cooked through. If not, return them to the pot for another 5 minutes or so, until they are cooked through.) Place on a cutting board and allow to cool to the touch.

4 Add rice, apples: Add the rice and the chopped apples to the soup. Return to a simmer on high heat, then lower the heat to maintain a low simmer. Cover and cook for 15 minutes, or until the rice is cooked through.

5 Shred the chicken, return to soup, add cream: While the apples and rice are cooking in the soup, shred the chicken, discarding any tough bits. Once the rice and apples in the soup are cooked, add the chicken back to the pot. Heat for 5 minutes more. Then stir in the cream.

Classic English Toad-in-the-Hole

INGREDIENTS

- 1 1/2 cup (180 g) of all purpose flour

- 1/2 teaspoon salt

- Pinch of freshly ground black pepper

- 3 eggs, beaten

- 1 1/2 cup (350 ml) milk

- 2 tablespoons melted butter

- 1 tablespoon vegetable oil

- 1 pound (450 g) of bangers (an English sausage made with pork and breadcrumbs), or good quality pork or beef sausage links (in casings)

METHODHIDE PHOTOS

1 Make batter: In a large bowl, whisk together the flour with the salt and a pinch of pepper. Make a well in the center of the flour. Pour in the eggs, milk, and melted butter into the well and whisk into the flour until smooth. Cover and let stand 30 minutes.

2 Pre-heat baking dish: Coat the bottom and sides of an 8x12 or 9x9 ceramic or metal casserole dish with vegetable oil. Place a rack in the bottom third of the oven. Put the empty dish on the rack. Preheat the oven with the dish in it to 425°F(220°C).

3 Brown the sausages: While the oven is coming to temperature, heat a tablespoon of vegetable oil in a skillet on medium high. Add the sausages and brown them on at least a couple sides.

4 Pour batter over sausages: When the sausages have browned, and the dish in the oven hot, pull the oven rack out a bit, put the sausages in the casserole dish, and pour the batter over the sausages.

5 Bake: Bake at 425°F(220°C) for about 20-30 minutes or until the batter is risen and golden.

Portuguese Salt Cod Stew (Bacalao or Bacalhoada)

INGREDIENTS

- 1 pound salt cod fillets, preferably skinless and boneless

- 3/4 to 1 cup of good quality extra virgin olive oil

- Milk (optional)

- 2 large yellow or sweet Vidalia onions, sliced

- 2 pounds waxy potatoes (Yukon gold work great), peeled

- 4 eggs, hard boiled and sliced

- About 40 pitted black olives (I used Kalamata olives, can also use green olives)

- Kosher salt and freshly ground black pepper

METHODHIDE PHOTOS

1 Soak salt cod in water: Salt cod typically comes either in dry fillets, already boned and skinned, or it comes whole. The fillets need to be rinsed, then soaked in water, and kept chilled, for 24 hours, with one or two changes of the water.

bacalao salt cod for bacalhoada portuguese stewbacalao salt cod soaking in water

If you are using a whole fish, not prepared fillets, it needs to be soaked in water for up to 48 hours, also with several changes of water, and the bones and the skin removed and discarded after soaking.

2 Simmer salt cod in milk and/or water: Put salt cod in a saucepan. Add enough milk, water, or a mixture of milk and water to just cover. Bring mixture to a simmer. Let simmer for a couple minutes. Remove the fish and set aside.

3 Parboil potatoes and slice: Parboil the potatoes for 20 minutes (you can cook them in the water you used to cook the fish if you want). Slice potatoes into 1/4-inch thick rounds.

4 Layer casserole with onions, potatoes, salt cod, olive oil, pepper, then top with hard boiled eggs and olives: In a large pyrex casserole or Dutch oven (use Dutch oven if making on stove-top), generously coat the bottom of the pan with olive oil. Place a layer of onion rings over the bottom of the pan.

Place a layer of sliced potatoes over the onions.

layer bacalao stew casserole with onions layer portuguese bacalhoada salt cod stew with potatoes

Breaking up the salt cod with your fingers, place pieces of salt cod in a layer over the potatoes. Taste the fish for saltiness. After a day of soaking and further cooking, there should be just a hint of saltiness in the fish. If most of the salt was soaked out of the fish, and the fish doesn't taste at all salty, you may need to sprinkle some salt back on to the fish as you place the layers down.

Generously pour some olive oil over the fish. Sprinkle with freshly grated black pepper.

layer bacaloa in the portuguese salt cod stewtop bacalao stew with eggs and olives

Repeat with another layer of onions, potatoes, fish, olive oil, pepper (and more salt if needed).

Then finish with layers of onions, potatoes, more olive oil, sliced hard boiled eggs, and olives.

5 Cook on stovetop or bake: Place on stove top on medium heat, and cook, covered, for 30 minutes. Or heat an oven to 350°F and cook, covered, for 30-40 minutes, or until everything is completely through.

Brazilian Salmon Stew (Moqueca)

INGREDIENTS

- Marinade:

- The cloves from 1/2 head of garlic, peeled, crushed, minced

- 2 Tablespoons of fresh lime juice

- 3/4 teaspoon of coarse salt

- 1 Tablespoon of sweet paprika

- 2 1/2 teaspoons of ground cumin

- 1 1/2 teaspoons of freshly ground black pepper

- Other:

- 1 1/2 to 2 pounds of salmon, cut into 2-inch pieces (largish-bite sized pieces)

- Extra virgin olive oil

- 2 medium onions, sliced

- 1 large green bell pepper, seeded, de-stemmed, and sliced

- 2 medium tomatoes, sliced

- Salt and freshly ground pepper

- 1 14-ounce can regular (not light) coconut milk

- 1 large bunch fresh cilantro, chopped, 1-2 cups

METHODHIDE PHOTOS

1 Marinate salmon: Mix together the marinade ingredients. Let the salmon marinate in this paste for at least 2 hours. The longer, the better.

2 Layer ingredients in a large pot: In a large pan (large covered skillet or Dutch oven), coat the bottom of the pan with a couple tablespoons of olive oil. Add a layer of sliced onions, and then a layer of sliced bell peppers, and a layer of sliced tomatoes.

Place the fish pieces, with the marinade, on top of everything, and start layering again—onions, bell peppers, and tomatoes.

3 Top with cilantro, coconut milk, olive oil: Sprinkle generously with salt and pepper. Add about half of your fresh cilantro to the top.

Pour coconut milk over the top. Drizzle generously with olive oil over the top (several tablespoons).

4 Simmer: Bring to a boil, reduce heat to low, cover and let simmer for 30 minutes to an hour, until the vegetables are cooked through.

Moqueca – Brazilian Fish Stew

INGREDIENTS

- Soup

- 1 1/2 to 2 pounds of fillets of firm white fish such as halibut, swordfish, or cod, rinsed in cold water, pin bones removed, cut into large portions

- 3 cloves garlic, minced

- 4 tablespoons lime or lemon juice

- Salt

- Freshly ground black pepper

- Extra virgin olive oil

- 1 cup chopped spring onion, or 1 medium yellow onion, chopped or sliced

- 1/4 cup green onion greens, chopped

- 1/2 yellow and 1/2 red bell pepper, seeded, de-stemmed, chopped (or sliced)

- 2 cups chopped (or sliced) tomatoes

- 1 tablespoon paprika (Hungarian sweet)

- Pinch red pepper flakes

- 1 large bunch of cilantro, chopped with some set aside for garnish

- 1 14-ounce can coconut milk

- Rice

- 1 tablespoon extra virgin olive oil

- 1/2 onion, chopped

- 1 clove garlic, minced

- 1 cup white rice

- 1 3/4 cups boiling water (check your rice package for the appropriate ratio of liquid to rice for the type of rice you are using)

- 1 teaspoon salt

METHODHIDE PHOTOS

1 Coat fish with garlic and lime juice: Place fish pieces in a bowl, add the minced garlic and lime juice so that the pieces are well coated. Sprinkle generously all over with salt and pepper.

Keep chilled while preparing the rest of the soup.

2 Make rice for serving with soup: If you are planning on serving the soup with rice, start on the rice.

Bring a couple cups of water to a boil. Heat one Tbsp of olive oil in a medium saucepan on medium high heat. Add the chopped 1/2 onion and cook, stirring, until the onion is translucent. Add the garlic and cook for 30 seconds more, until the garlic is fragrant. Add the raw white rice and stir to coat completely with the oil, onions, and garlic.

Add the boiling water. (The amount depends on your brand of rice, check the package. If no amounts are given, add 1 3/4 cup of water for every cup of rice.) Stir in 1 teaspoon of salt.

Bring to a simmer, then lower the heat, cover, and let cook for 15 minutes, after which, remove from heat until ready to serve with the soup.

3 Start cooking the onion, bell pepper, tomatoes, onion greens: In a large covered pan (such as a

Dutch oven), coat the bottom with about 2 Tbsp of olive oil and heat on medium heat.

Add the chopped onion and cook a few minutes until softened. Add the bell pepper, paprika, and red pepper flakes. Sprinkle generously with salt and pepper. (At least a teaspoon of salt.) Cook for a few minutes longer, until the bell pepper begins to soften.

Stir in the chopped tomatoes and onion greens. Bring to a simmer and cook for 5 minutes, uncovered. Stir in the chopped cilantro.

4 Layer vegetables with fish, add coconut milk: Use a large spoon to remove about half of the vegetables (you'll put them right back in). Spread the remaining vegetables over the bottom of the pan to create a bed for the fish.

Arrange the fish pieces on the vegetables. Sprinkle with salt and pepper. Then add back the previously removed vegetables, covering the fish.

Pour coconut milk over the fish and vegetables.

5 Simmer, cook, adjust seasonings: Bring soup to a simmer, reduce the heat, cover, and let

simmer for 15 minutes. Taste and adjust seasonings.

You may need to add more salt (likely), lime or lemon juice, paprika, pepper, or chili flakes to get the soup to the desired seasoning for your taste.

Garnish with cilantro. Serve with rice or with crusty bread.

INGREDIENTS

- 1 large egg*

- 1/3 cup extra virgin olive oil

- 2/3 cup milk

- 1 1/2 cups (170 grams) tapioca flour

- 1/2 cup (packed, about 66 grams) grated cheese, your preference, we get good results with feta cheese (no need to grate), or fresh farmer's cheese (if using fresh farmer's cheese, you may want to add another 1/2 teaspoon of salt)
- 1 teaspoon of salt (or more to taste)
- mini-muffin-tin.jpg

- *It helps when baking with eggs to start with eggs at room temperature. If you don't plan ahead (that would be me, usually) you can put the egg in a bowl of warm water for a few minutes to gently take off the chill of the fridge.

- Special equipment:

- One 24-well or or two 12-well mini muffin tins. Mini muffin tins are about half the size of a regular muffin pan. The muffin openings are about 1-inch deep, and 1 3/4 inch wide at the top.

METHODSHOW PHOTOS

1 Pre-heat oven, prepare mini-muffin tin: Preheat oven to 400°F. Spread a small amount olive oil around the insides of each well of a mini-muffin tin.

2 Blend ingredients: Put all of the ingredients into a blender and pulse until smooth. You may need to use a spatula to scrape down the sides of the blender so that everything gets blended well. At this point you can store the batter in the refrigerator for up to a week.

3 Pour into mini-muffin tin: Pour batter into prepared mini-muffin tin, not quite to the top; leave about 1/8 inch from the top.

4 Bake: Bake at 400°F in the oven for 15-20 minutes, until all puffy and nicely browned. Remove from oven and let cool on a rack for a few minutes.

Eat while warm or save to reheat later.

Note that Brazilian cheese bread is very chewy, a lot like Japanese mochi.

Yeasted Belgian Waffles Recipe

INGREDIENTS

- For the waffle batter:

- 1 3/4 cups whole milk

- 2 1/4 teaspoon (7g) active yeast (or 1 package, not fast acting or instant)

- 2 cups (280g) all-purpose flour

- 1/4 cup (40g) yellow cornmeal

- 1 tablespoon brown sugar
- 1 teaspoon kosher salt
- 1/2 cup unsalted butter, melted
- 2 large eggs
- 1/2 teaspoon baking soda
- For topping:

- Powdered sugar, optional
- Maple syrup
- Whipped cream
- Fresh fruit
- Jam or preserves of your choice
- Special equipment:

- Belgian Waffle Iron

METHOD SHOW PHOTOS

1 Make the batter: Warm the milk up on the stovetop until it is warm to the touch, but not hot. (This should only take about 5 to 10 seconds on a gas or induction stovetop; an electric will take slightly longer.) Remove from heat and pour into a large mixing bowl. Add the yeast and stir to dissolve. Let the mixture sit for 5 minutes to proof. You should see a few bubbles form at the top.

Add the flour, cornmeal, brown sugar, and salt to the yeasted milk. Stir with a large spatula, and as the dry ingredients become incorporated into the batter, drizzle the melted butter over the entire mixture, stirring constantly. Stir until all the dry ingredients are absorbed and then cover the bowl with plastic wrap.

2 Let the batter sit on the counter overnight, up to 8 hours.

3 The next day, preheat your waffle iron. Spray your waffle iron lightly with cooking oil.

Also, preheat your oven to 250°F for the finished waffles. Place a wire metal rack on a rimmed baking sheet and put in the oven—or directly onto the oven rack itself.

4 Make the waffles: The batter will have more than doubled in size after resting. Whisk in the eggs and baking soda. This will deflate the batter.

Pour 3/4 cup (or the manufacturer's suggested amount) of batter into the waffle maker, making sure it fills all the crevices. Close and cook the waffle to your preferred toasty level.

5 Keep the waffles warm until serving: Once the waffle is done, move the waffle to the warm oven, on the wire racked baking sheet and repeat the process until all the batter is used and waffles made. Serve with a dusting of powdered sugar, maple syrup on the side, or whatever topping you choose!

Rabbit Braised in Belgian Ale

INGREDIENTS

- One 2 1/2 to 3 pound rabbit, cut into 6 to 7 serving pieces (2 front legs, 2 back legs, the loin cut into 2 to 3 pieces), plus ribs and flap meat

- Salt

- 1/2 cup all purpose flour for dredging

- 2 tablespoons extra virgin olive oil

- 2 tablespoons butter

- 2 medium onions, sliced stem to root (about 2 1/2 cups sliced)

- 4-6 whole cloves of garlic, peeled

- 6 sprigs of fresh thyme, tied together with kitchen string (or 1/2 teaspoon dried thyme)

- 1 1/2 cups of Belgian ale, such as Chimay or Ommengang

- 1/2 cup of chicken stock

- 1/2 teaspoon salt

- 1/2 teaspoon freshly ground black pepper

- 1 celery root, peeled and diced

- 2 teaspoons whole grained mustard

- 2 teaspoons brown sugar

- 1 tablespoon chopped fresh parsley

METHODSHOW PHOTOS

1 Sprinkle rabbit pieces with salt: Place rabbit pieces on a platter, sprinkle both sides with kosher salt. Let sit for 30 minutes to an hour.

2 Dredge rabbit with flour, brown in butter: Place flour on plate. Dredge rabbit pieces in flour.

Heat oil and butter in a large Dutch oven on medium heat (large enough to fit rabbit pieces in a single layer). Once the butter is melted and foamy, add the rabbit pieces in a single layer to the pot.

Brown on one side without stirring for 5 to 6 minutes. Then turn the pieces over and brown on the other side. Remove to a plate.

3 Brown the onions, add garlic and thyme: Add the sliced onions to the pot, and cook, stirring occasionally, until lightly brown, scraping up and browned rabbit bits from the bottom of the pot. Add garlic cloves and thyme, cook until onions are soft and the garlic quite fragrant.

4 Add ale, then stock, salt, pepper: Increase the heat to high and add the Belgian ale. Let it simmer for a minute or two, then add the stock. Add a half teaspoon of salt and the freshly ground black pepper.

5 Add celery root, rabbit, then simmer: Place the diced celery root over the onions in a single layer. Place the browned rabbit pieces over the celery root. Bring to a simmer. Cover and reduce heat to maintain a very low simmer. Cook for 45 minutes, or until the rabbit is just cooked through and tender.

6 Reduce sauce: Remove rabbit pieces from the pot and keep warm on a platter. Increase the heat to high and reduce the liquid by one third. Then, reduce the heat to low, stir in the mustard and sugar. Taste and add more salt and pepper in needed.

7 Return meat to sauce in pot: Slice the flap meat pieces of the rabbit into strips and return to the pot. Strip away any available meat from the back and chest parts and return meat to the pot. Add the serving pieces to the pot. Cover and let rewarm for a minute.

8 Serve: Sprinkle with chopped parsley to serve. Serve with crusty bread, egg noodles, or rice pilaf, along with some Belgian ale.

Winter Chicken Salad with Tangy Miso Dressing

INGREDIENTS

- For the salad

- 1 pound boneless skinless chicken breasts

- Kosher salt

- Freshly ground black pepper

- 1 head butter lettuce, washed and dried

- 1 large handful arugula or watercress, washed and dried

- 1 small or 1/2 large bulb fennel, very thinly sliced

- 3 seedless mandarins, peeled, cut into wheels, and pulled into pieces

- 1 small avocado, diced

- For the miso dressing

- 1/4 cup plus 2 teaspoons extra-virgin olive oil

- 1 tablespoon white miso paste

- 1 tablespoon plus 2 teaspoons apple cider vinegar

- 1 teaspoon honey

- 2 scallions, white and light green parts only, finely chopped
- 1/2 teaspoon ground cumin
- Special equipment:
- Meat pounder or rolling pin

METHOD SHOW PHOTOS

1 Pound the chicken: Lay the chicken breasts on a cutting board. Use a mallet or the side of a rolling pin to pound the thicker end of the breasts, so they're about the same thickness along the whole breast. Season on both sides with salt and freshly ground pepper.

2 Cook the chicken: Heat 2 teaspoons of the olive oil over medium in a large cast-iron or non-stick skillet. Cook the chicken until nicely browned on one side and opaque halfway up the side, about 8 minutes.

Flip and cook on the second side until no longer pink in the center, another 8 minutes or so. Transfer to a cutting board to rest for at least 5 minutes. Cut across the grain in 1/3-inch-thick slices.

3 Make the miso dressing: In a small bowl, whisk together the miso, apple cider vinegar, honey, scallions, and cumin until smooth. Continue to whisk as you drizzle in the remaining olive oil.

4 Assemble the salad: Toss the lettuce, arugula, and fennel in a large bowl with just enough dressing to lightly coat. Transfer to 4 serving bowls. Tuck the avocado, mandarins, and chicken slices into the bowls and dribble a little more dressing over them. Serve immediately.

Teriyaki Chicken Breasts

INGREDIENTS

- 3/4 cup soy sauce* (or mix tamari** and water in equal proportions to make 3/4 cup)

- 3/4 cup sake

- 3/4 cup mirin

- 4 Tbsp sugar

- A 1-inch piece of ginger, grated fine

- 4 skinless, boneless chicken breasts, about 1 1/4 to 1 1/2 pounds total (set out for 30 minutes to come to room temp)

- 2-3 Tbsp sesame seeds

- *Use gluten-free soy sauce for gluten-free version.

- **If you are using tamari instead of soy sauce, use half as much, as tamari is more concentrated than soy sauce.

METHOD

1 Gently simmer chicken in sauce made with sake, mirin, soy sauce, sugar, ginger: Mix the grated ginger, sugar, soy sauce, sake and mirin in a pot and bring to a boil. Add the chicken breasts, return to a simmer, then lower the heat to the lowest possible setting (warm if you can), on your smallest burner, and cover.

The idea is to cook the chicken as gently as possible, below a simmer. Cook for 20 minutes.

If you are working with somewhat large chicken breasts, you may need to cook them longer, or cut them in half before cooking.

2 Toast sesame seeds: While the chicken is poaching, toast the sesame seeds in a dry pan until they begin to brown. Move to a small bowl and set aside.

3 Set aside chicken, cover with foil: Remove the chicken breasts from the teriyaki sauce, set on a plate and wrap with foil.

4 Reduce sauce: Bring the sauce back to a boil and boil vigorously until the sauce is reduced to a syrup, about 8-10 minutes. Keep an eye on the sauce, stirring it occasionally.

5 Slice chicken, cover with sauce, sprinkle with sesame seeds and serve: To serve, slice the chicken breasts, cover with the teriyaki sauce and sprinkle sesame seeds on them. Serve with plain white rice.

Miso Glazed Salmon

INGREDIENTS

- 2 Tbsp red miso or 3 Tbsp white miso

- 2 Tbsp sake

- 2 Tbsp sugar (less or more to taste)

- 2 teaspoons soy sauce

- 4 6-ounce skinless salmon fillets

METHODSHOW PHOTOS

1 Mix the miso, sake, soy sauce, and sugar in a small bowl. Adjust proportions to taste.

2 Marinate the salmon: Pour half of the mixture into a container large enough to fit the salmon fillets, then pour the rest over the top of the fish. Make sure the fish is coated with the miso sauce.

Cover the container and marinate for at least 30 minutes, and up to overnight.

3 Broil the salmon: Line a broiling pan with aluminum foil. Brush a little vegetable oil over

the foil and lay the salmon fillets on top. Make sure there is an even, thin coating of marinade on top of the fish.

Place the fillets no closer than about 6 inches from the broiler element in your oven. Broil for 6-10 minutes, depending on how thick the fillets are and how hot your broiler is.

Keep an eye on the salmon. The marinade has sugar in it that can easily cause the glaze to burn. If it starts charring and the cooking isn't yet finished, place the fish on a lower rack in the oven.

Serve with rice and stir-fried vegetables.

Easy Weeknight Chicken Ramen

INGREDIENTS

- For the broth:

- 2 tablespoons toasted sesame oil

- 4 scallions, thinly sliced, including some of the green part

- 1 clove garlic, minced

- 1 small carrot, peeled and thinly sliced

- 4 ounces button, cremini, or shiitake mushrooms, thinly sliced

- 1 1/2 cups thinly shredded Napa cabbage, spinach, kale, or other greens

- 1-inch piece fresh ginger, minced

- 6 cups low-sodium chicken broth, store-bought or homemade

- 1 tablespoon brown sugar, optional

- Lime wedges, optional

- For the soup:

- 4 large eggs

- 20 ounces fresh ramen noodles, or 12 ounces dried noodles

- 2 medium cooked chicken breast halves, sliced (see Recipe Note)

- For the garnish:

- Soy sauce

- Sriracha or other hot sauce

- Handful fresh cilantro, leaves removed from stems

- Lime wedges

METHODSHOW PHOTOS

1 Make the broth: In a large saucepan over medium heat, heat the oil. Add the scallions, garlic, carrot, mushrooms, and cabbage. Cook, stirring often, for 3 minutes, or until the vegetables soften.

Stir in the ginger and brown sugar (if using) and cook for 30 seconds. Finally add the chicken broth and bring to a simmer. Simmer for 10 minutes.

2 Cook the eggs: While the broth is simmering, bring a pot of water to a boil. Set a bowl of cold ice water nearby.

Use a slotted spoon to gently lower the eggs, still in the shell, into the water. Simmer for 7 minutes for eggs that are soft and a little runny in the center, or 9 minutes for hard-boiled eggs.

Transfer the eggs to the bowl of cold water and set aside until ready to serve.

3 Cook the noodles: Return the pot of water to a boil. Add the noodles and cook for 3 minutes, or according to the package directions, until tender. Drain in a colander.

4 Assemble the soup: Divide the noodles among 4 large bowls. Ladle the broth and vegetables over the noodles.

Remove the eggs from the ice water. Tap the shells with a spoon to crack and then peel off the shells. Pat the eggs dry and cut them in half.

Top each bowl with the egg halves and the sliced chicken. Serve with soy sauce, hot sauce, cilantro leaves and lime wedges.

Pan Simmered Pacific Black Cod

INGREDIENTS

- 1 to 1 1/2 pounds black cod fillets, skin on or skinless

- 1/4 cup sake

- 1/4 cup rice vinegar

- 1/4 cup canola, rice bran or other neutral oil

- 2 Tbsp soy sauce

- 1 Tbsp minced fresh ginger

- Dark sesame oil, for garnish

- 3 green onions, thinly sliced on the diagonal, for garnish

- 1 Tbsp toasted sesame seeds, for garnish

METHOD

1 Prepare sauce: In a large sauté pan, mix the sake, rice vinegar, canola oil, soy sauce and ginger. Bring to a simmer on medium to medium high heat.

2 Simmer fish in sauce: Lay each fillet in the pan. (If using skin-on fillets, place the fillets skin-side down in the pan.) Use a spoon to baste the tops of each fillet until you see the flakes of

the fish separate a little, which should take about 30 seconds to 1 minute per fillet.

Let the fish simmer for 3-6 minutes, depending on how thick they are. Estimate 3 minutes for a 1/4 inch-thick fillet, up to 6 minutes for an inch-thick fillet.

Gently move the fish to individual plates. If you want, use (clean) needle-nosed pliers or tweezers to remove the pin bones in the fillets.

3 Reduce sauce: Increase the heat on the sauce and boil vigorously for 1 minute, stirring constantly to reduce the sauce.

4 Serve: Spoon a tablespoon or more of the sauce over each fillet and discard the rest. Drizzle a little bit of sesame oil over each fillet, then garnish with the green onions and toasted sesame seeds. Serve immediately.

Tempura Fried Calamari

INGREDIENTS

- 1 pound cleaned squid

- 1 egg yolk

- 1 cup ice cold sparkling water (the colder the better)

- 1/8 teaspoon baking soda

- 1 teaspoon salt

- 1/4 cup cornstarch

- 3/4 cup rice or regular flour plus more for sprinkling on squid

- Peanut oil or canola oil for frying

- Special equipment:

- A deep fryer

METHOD

1 Slice the squid tubes into rings: Slice the squid tubes into rings about 1/2-inch to 3/4-inch wide. Leave the tentacles whole.

2 Heat oil in a deep fryer or large heavy pot: This recipe was designed for a deep-fryer, but

you can also fill a large, heavy-bottomed pot (keep a lid nearby, for safety reasons) halfway with oil, about 3 inches deep. Heat the oil to 360-370°F.

3 Mix dry ingredients: While the oil is heating, mix all the dry ingredients together well.

4 Mix sparkling water with egg yolk, then mix with dry ingredients: Once the oil has reached 360°F, take the sparkling water out of the refrigerator and mix it with the egg yolk. Immediately mix it in with the dry ingredients.

Mix quickly. Do not worry if there are clumps or lumps. Over-mixing may cause the batter to become chewy when cooked.

5 Sprinkle squid pieces with flour. Use a small sieve to lightly dust the squid pieces with rice flour or regular flour. This will help the batter adhere to the squid.

6 Dip squid pieces in batter and fry in hot oil: Working in small batches at a time (about 6 pieces), dip the squid pieces in the batter. Pick them up one by one and gently put them in the hot oil. (Note if your fingers are coated with the batter, it will help protect them from splatter.)

When the squid pieces are in the oil, use a chopstick or the handle of a wooden spoon to dislodge any squid pieces that may have become stuck from the bottom of the pot or fryer. Fry for 45 seconds to 1 minute, and remove to paper towels to drain.

Note that when done, they will NOT be golden brown, but more of a pale yellow or tan.

Repeat with the rest of the squid. Working in batches will help keep the oil temperature from falling too far while you are frying the squid.

6 Serve immediately: Serve immediately with lime or lemon wedges, soy sauce, ponzu sauce, Tabasco or another hot sauce.

Once the cooking oil has completely cooled (after about 2 hours), strain it through a paper towel-lined sieve, and save it to reuse the next time you want to deep fry seafood.

Seared Ahi Tuna

INGREDIENTS

- 2 (6-8 ounce) ahi tuna steaks (3/4 of an inch thick)
- For the marinade:

- 2 tablespoons dark sesame oil

- 2 tablespoons soy sauce (or 2 teaspoons of wheat-free tamari for gluten-free option)

- 1 tablespoon of grated fresh ginger

- 1 clove garlic, minced

- 1 green onion (scallion) thinly sliced (a few slices reserved for garnish)

- 1 teaspoon lime juice

METHOD

1 Marinate the tuna steaks: Mix the marinade ingredients together and coat the tuna steaks with the marinade, cover tightly, and refrigerate for at least an hour.

2 Sear the tuna: Heat a non-stick skillet over medium high to high heat. When the pan is hot, remove the tuna steaks from the marinade and sear them for a minute to a minute and a half on each side (even a little longer if you want the tuna less rare than pictured.)

3 Slice and serve: Remove from pan and slice into 1/4-inch thick slices. Sprinkle with a few green onion slices.

Serve plain, with white rice, or over lettuce or thinly sliced cabbage or fennel. Shown served over sliced fennel salad.

Ambrosia Salad

INGREDIENTS

- 1 cup shredded sweetened coconut, toasted
- 1 (15 oz) can mandarin oranges, drained
- 1 (15 oz) can pineapple chunks, drained
- 1/2 cup maraschino cherries, halved
- 3 cups mini marshmallows
- 1 apple, peeled and chopped (any kind will do)
- 1/4 cup slivered almonds
- For the whipped cream dressing:
- 1 cup heavy whipping cream
- 1/4 cup sour cream

- 2 tablespoons sugar

METHOD

1 Toast the coconut: Add coconut to a dry medium skillet set over medium-low heat. Toast until fragrant, stirring regularly. Watch it closely, as it can burn quickly. When the coconut starts to turn a light brown color, 2 to 3 minutes, it's done.

This is an optional step, but it gives a flavor boost to the coconut.

2 Mixing the salad: Add the toasted coconut to a bowl with the orange segments, pineapple

chunks, cherries, mini marshmallows, apples, and almonds. Stir together well.

3 Make the whipped cream dressing: In a stand mixer fitted with the whisk attachment, or with a hand mixer, beat heavy whipping cream on high for 2 to 3 minutes until it starts to stiffen.

Then add the sour cream and sugar, and continue to whip until the mixture is still silky but holds firm peaks. Do not overwhip.

4 Finish the salad: Fold the whipped cream mixture into the fruit and nut mixture.

5 Serve: Serve immediately. Keep the ambrosia salad leftovers in the fridge for up two days.

Apple and Sweet Potato Matzo Bake

INGREDIENTS

- 6 large eggs
- 1/2 teaspoon salt
- 1/2 teaspoon ground black pepper
- 2 cups hot water
- 6 sheets (6 ounces) matzo crackers, broken into 1-inch pieces
- 1 1/2 pounds sweet potatoes, peeled and sliced into 1/8-inch-thick rounds
- 2 large Fuji or gala apples, peeled, quartered, cored, and sliced into 1/4-inch-thick slices
- 1 teaspoon cinnamon
- 2 tablespoons margarine

METHOD

1 Preheat oven and prepare baking dish: Preheat the oven to 325º F. Grease a 9x13 baking dish with margarine, olive oil, or grapeseed oil.

2 Beat the eggs and soak the matzo: In a medium bowl, beat the eggs, salt, and pepper until no streaks of yolk remain.

In separate large bowl, pour the hot water over the matzo crackers. Let sit for just a minute. Drain the excess water.

3 Add the eggs mixture to the matzo: Pour the egg mixture over the drained matzo and gently

fold to combine. You don't want to break up or smush the matzo pieces too much, just coat them evenly in egg.

4 Layer the potatoes and apples: Place half of the sweet potato slices in the baking dish in an even layer. Place half of the apple slices on top of the sweet potatoes, then sprinkle 1/2 teaspoon of the cinnamon over the apples. Spoon half of the matzo/egg mixture over the apples and spread it out in an even layer.

Repeat the layers of sweet potato, apple, cinnamon, and matzo/egg mixture once more, then cover the dish with aluminum foil, making sure the foil isn't touching the matzo.

5 Bake the casserole and dot with margarine: Bake the casserole, covered, for 1 hour. Remove from the oven, uncover, and poke with a paring knife or toothpick to make sure the sweet potatoes are softened and cooked through. (If they aren't soft yet, re-cover the casserole and bake for another 10 minutes, or until the sweet potatoes are soft enough to easily pierce.)

Dot the top of the casserole with margarine and bake, uncovered, for another 5 minutes, until the margarine is melted and the matzo is lightly browned.

6 Cool and cut: Remove the matzo bake from the oven, let stand for 15 minutes, then cut into slices and serve warm.

Charoset with Apples, Dates, and Walnuts

INGREDIENTS

- 1 cup walnut halves and pieces

- 1/2 pound (about 13 large) medjool dates, pitted

- 1/4 cup orange juice or Manischewitz wine

- 1 Granny Smith or Fuji apple, peeled, cored, and chopped

- 1/2 teaspoon cinnamon

- 1/4 teaspoon ginger

METHOD

1 Process the nuts: Add the walnuts to a food processor. Process them in 1-second pulses, until they are finely chopped. Transfer them to a bowl. Reserve 1 tablespoon to use as a garnish.

2 Create a paste: Add the pitted dates and orange juice to the now-empty food processor. Process them until they form a thick paste, scraping down the sides if necessary.

3 Combine the ingredients: Add the paste to the bowl with the chopped nuts. Add the apple,

cinnamon, and ginger to the bowl and stir to combine.

4 Adjust the flavor and serve: Taste the charoset and add more juice or wine, cinnamon, or ginger to taste. The charoset can be served right away, or up to two days after it is prepared. (Keep refrigerated.) To garnish, sprinkle with the reserved tablespoon of walnuts.

Apple Galette with Blue Cheese, Almonds and Honey

INGREDIENTS

- For the dough:

- 1 cup (130g) all-purpose flour

- 2 tablespoons sugar

- 1/2 teaspoon salt

- 1/2 cup (113g) cold, unsalted butter, cut into small cubes

- 3 tablespoons ice water

- For the filling:

- 3 medium (about 1 pound) baking apples, such as Honeycrisp, Macoun or Empire,

- 1/4 teaspoon nutmeg

- 3 tablespoons turbinado sugar or sugar-in-the-raw

- 3 tablespoons sliced almonds

- 2 tablespoons crumbled blue cheese

- 2 tablespoons honey

METHOD

1 Chill the ingredients for the pie crust: In a mixing bowl, stir the flour, sugar and salt until combined. Add the butter cubes and toss to coat them in the flour. Place in the freezer for 20 minutes while you prepare the apples.

2 Prepare the apples: Cut the apples in half and slice out the cores, leaving the peels on. With the flat sides down, cut the apple halves into 3/8-inch-thick half-moon slices.

3 Make the pie crust: Transfer the chilled flour and butter mixture to the bowl of a food processor. Pulse in short bursts until the butter is cut into pea-size pieces. (A few large pieces are okay.)

Open the top of the food processor and drizzle the ice water over the mixture. Replace the lid and pulse again in short bursts until the mixture looks uniform and crumbly but does not yet form large clumps of dough.

Press a small amount of the dough together in your hand. It should form a clump that holds together firmly when pressed without cracking at the edges. If it feels crumbly or dry, sprinkle with additional ice water, 1 tablespoon at a time, and pulse briefly to mix.

4 Chill the pie crust: Turn out the crumbly dough onto the countertop. Press the dough into a flat disk with the palms of your hands without manipulating it too much. Wrap it in plastic wrap and refrigerate for 15 to 20 minutes.

5 Preheat the oven to 425F. Line a baking sheet with parchment.

6 Roll out the pie crust: On a floured work surface with a floured rolling pin, roll the dough

into a 12-inch circle. Transfer to the parchment-lined baking sheet.

7 Fill and bake the tart: Leaving a 2-inch border all around and starting at the outer edge, overlap the apple slices to fill the pie crust. Sprinkle with the nutmeg and sugar. Fold the edge of the pie crust over the apples.

8 Bake for 30 minutes, or until the apples are tender and the crust is golden.

9 Toast the almonds: While the tart is baking, spread the almonds on a baking sheet and toast

in the oven for 3 to 5 minutes, until golden. Watch carefully to keep them from burning.

10 Finish the tart: Remove the tart from the oven. Sprinkle with the toasted almonds and blue cheese crumbles. Drizzle the honey over top. Cut into wedges and serve.

Gruyere, Apple, and Fig Jam Panini

INGREDIENTS

- 2 Tbsp butter, at room temperature to make it easy to spread

- 4 slices rustic whole-grain bread, sliced from a dense bakery loaf

- 2 Tbsp fig jam

- 4 ounces Gruyere cheese, thinly sliced

- 1/2 Granny Smith apple, cored and thinly sliced

METHOD

1 Heat the panini press to medium-high heat. (Or if not using a panini press, preheat a cast iron frying pan on medium high heat.)

2 Assemble sandwiches: For each sandwich, spread butter on two slices of bread. Turn the slices over and spread a layer of fig jam on the other side of each slice.

To one slice add a layer of sliced cheese, several apple slices, and a layer of more cheese. Top the sandwich with the other slice of bread, buttered side up.

3 Grill in panini press: Place up to two panini at a time in the preheated panini maker, and close the lid closed. Grill until the cheese is melted and the bread is toasted, about 4 to 5 minutes.

Vegan Sweet Potatoes

INGREDIENTS

- Medium Sized Sweet Potatoes

- Agave Sweetener

- 3 Tablespoons Cinnamon

- 1 Teaspoon Nutmeg

INSTRUCTIONS

1. Preheat oven to 400 degrees.

2. Cut sweet potato in chunks

3. Evenly distribute in a baking dish.

4. Sprinkle cinnamon and nutmeg over sweet potatoes.

5. Add agave and water on top.

6. Repeat steps of adding sweeteners until all sweet potatoes are in the pan

7. Place in oven for 45 min to an hour (depending on how soft you want them).

8. Let cool and enjoy!

Thai Chicken

Ingredients

- 2 chicken fillets
- 2 tbsp chopped fresh coriander (cilantro)
- 1 red chilli, de-seeded and chopped small
- 1 egg
- 1 tbsp white rice flour
- 1 tbsp sesame seeds
- 1 tsp garlic-infused oil
- Salt and pepper to taste

For the dipping sauce

- 3 tbsp soy sauce

- 2 tbsp lemon juice

Method

1. Slice the chicken fillets in half horizontally to create 4 fillets.

2. Mix the next 7 ingredients in a shallow bowl.

3. Dip the chicken in the mixture and make sure they are well covered.

4. Heat some oil/butter in a frying pan and fry the chicken until just cooked through but with no pink left.

For the dipping sauce:

1. Mix the two ingredients together and serve in a small bowl for each person.

2. Serve with chips and a mixed salad.

Grilled Halibut with Fennel Sauce Recipe

Ingredients

- Grilled Halibut:

- 2 teaspoons fennel seeds

- 2 large garlic cloves, minced

- 1 lemon, juiced

- 1 teaspoon coarse salt

- 2 tablespoons olive oil, extra-virgin

- 8 (1-inch thick) halibut steaks (about 3/4 pound each)*

- Fennel Sauce:

- 1 medium fennel bulb with fronds (about 3/4 pound)

- 1 teaspoon fennel seeds

- 2 garlic cloves, minced

- 1 lemon, juiced

Instructions

Grilled Halibut Instructions:

Prepare Fennel Sauce (see recipe below); set aside. Preheat barbecue grill. Lightly oil the racks to keep halibut from sticking.

In a dry small frying pan over medium heat, toast fennel seeds, shaking pan, until fragrant and a shade darker. In an electric coffee/spice grinder grind the toasted fennel seeds.

In a small bowl, stir together lemon juice, ground fennel seeds, garlic, salt, and olive oil. Place halibut in a large dish and pour marinade over it, turning fish to coat. Marinate halibut, covered and refrigerated, at least 10 minutes and no more than 1 hour.

Remove halibut from marinade and discard marinade.

Cover barbecue with lid, open any vents, and grill halibut about 5 minutes on each side or until a meat thermometer registers an internal temperature of 140 degrees F (halibut will be slightly opaque in thickest part). Remember the halibut continues to cook after it is removed from the heat source.

Approximately cooking times for halibut:

1/4 to 1/3-inch - 3 to 4 minutes

12 to 3/4-inch - 4 to 6 minutes

1 to 1 1/2-inch - 8 to 12 minutes

Carefully remove the halibut from the grill and transfer onto individual serving plates.

Serve with Fennel Sauce.

Makes 8 servings.

Fennel Sauce Instructions:

Trim fennel stalks flush with bulb, reserving fronds and discarding stalks. Also trim off any discolored outer layers and discard. Halve bulb lengthwise and discard core. Finely chop fronds and bulb.

In a dry small frying pan, toast fennel seeds over moderate heat, shaking skillet, until fragrant and a shade darker. In an electric coffee/spice grinder grind seeds.

In a large bowl, combined chopped fennel, ground fennel seeds, garlic, yogurt, salt, and lemon juice to taste. NOTE: May be made 3 days ahead and refrigerated, covered.

Makes about 3 cups.

Truffle Custard with Crab and Caviar Recipe

Ingredients

- 2 eggs

- 1 egg yolk

- 1/2 teaspoon white Truffle Oil

- 2/3 cup heavy cream

- 1/3 cup milk

- 1 tablespoon soy sauce

- 1/2 pound Dungeness Crab Meat

- 1 tablespoon chives, finely chopped

- 2 teaspoons lime juice, freshly squeezed

- Salt and coarsely-ground black pepper, to taste

- 1/2 ounce caviar (hackleback or other black caviar)

Instructions

Preheat the oven to 325 degrees F. Adjust oven rack to center position.

Arrange 12 shot glasses in a 9-by-9-inch baking pan. Bring a kettle of water to a low simmer over low heat.

Meanwhile, in a medium bowl whisk together the eggs, egg yolk, and truffle oil; set aside.

In a small saucepan over medium heat, combine the cream, milk, and soy sauce. Bring just to a boil, stirring constantly; remove from the heat and let cool 1 minute. Whisking constantly, slowly pour the hot cream mixture into the eggs. Immediately strain the mixture through a mesh strainer into a large liquid measuring cup (or other container or pitcher with a pouring spout).

Carefully pour the strained custard mixture into the shot glasses, filling them about 3/4 full. Carefully pour enough hot water from the kettle into the baking pan to reach halfway up the shot glasses. Cover the pan with aluminum foil and bake approximately 9 to 10 minutes or until a knife inserted near the center comes out clean (the custards should be firm at the edges and just barely wobbly at the center). If needed, cook another 1 to 2 minutes.

Remove from oven and immediately remove cups from the water bath. Let cool at room temperature until ready to serve.

While the custards cook and cool, prepare the crab mixture. In a small bowl, gently mix together the crab, chives, and lime juice. Season with salt and pepper to taste.

To serve, spoon a small amount of the prepared crab mixture over each custard, then top with a dollop of caviar.

Makes 12 shot glasses.

Tomato-Basil Crab Bisque Recipe

Ingredients

- 2 tablespoons butter, unsalted
- 10 ounces crab meat (fresh or canned), divided*
- 1 tomato, peeled, seeded and chopped (about 1/2 cup)**
- 1/3 cup plus 3 tablespoons basil leaves, fresh, chopped
- 2 cloves garlic, minced
- 1/2 cup flour (all-purpose)
- 1 3/4 cups clam juice
- 1 (5.5-ounce) can V8 vegetable juice
- 1 cup whipping cream or heavy cream
- 1 to 2 teaspoons old bay seasoning
- 1/4 teaspoon hot pepper sauce

- 3/4 cup water

- 2 tablespoons lemon juice, freshly squeezed

- Salt and pepper to taste

Instructions

In a large heavy soup pot over low heat, melt butter. NOTE: I like to use low heat when making this soup, as it gives me more control.

Add 3/4 of the crab meat, chopped tomato, 1/3 cup chopped fresh basil, and garlic; saute 2 minutes.

Whisk in flour and stir for 2 minutes. Whisk in clam juice, V8 vegetable juice, whipping cream, Old Bay seasoning, and hot pepper sauce. Simmer over low heat until slightly thickened, approximately 10 to 15 minutes. Remove from heat and let soup cool slightly.

Puree soup in batches in a food processor or blender until smooth.

Return pureed soup to the pot pot. Stir in water and lemon juice. Season to taste with salt and pepper.

NOTE: Can be made 1 day ahead. Chill uncovered until cold, then cover and keep refrigerated.

Bring to a simmer before serving.

To serve, divide soup among 6 individual soup bowls. Sprinkle with remaining crabmeat and 3 tablespoons basil.

Makes 6 first-course servings.

Stuffed Snow Peas with Crab Recipe

Ingredients

- 1/2 pound snow peas, fresh

- 12 ounces crab meat, well drained

- 2 eggs, hard-cooked, finely chopped

- 1/4 cup mayonnaise, light (more if needed)

- 1/4 to 1/2 teaspoons horseradish, prepared, or to taste

- 3 dashes of hot sauce or to taste

- 2 teaspoons capers, drained and minced

- 3 tablespoons celery, finely chopped

Instructions

Wash and clean snow peas. Using a sharp knife, split the snow peas on top side, leaving bottom intact to form a little boat. Blanch in lightly salted boiling water for 10 seconds; remove from heat. Immediately submerge snow peas in cold water for a minute. Remove and drain; set aside to cool. NOTE: Do not over cook the pea pods or you will have soggy pods instead of a nice crisp bite.

In a medium bowl, add crab meat, eggs, mayonnaise, horseradish, hot sauce, capers, and celery; mix very gently so as not to break up crab meat.

Stuff cooled snow peas generously with crab meat filling (about 1 heaping teaspoonfuls of each snow pea). Chill in refrigerator until ready to serve.

Makes about 24 stuffed snow peas.

She Crab Soup History and Recipe

Ingredients

- Charleston She Crab Soup:

- 2 tablespoons butter, divided

- 2 tablespoons all-purpose flour

- 1 cup milk

- 1 1/2 cup half & half cream

- 4 teaspoons onion, finely grated

- 3/4 teaspoon Worcestershire sauce

- Salt and white pepper to taste

- 1/4 teaspoon mace, ground

- 1/4 teaspoon cayenne pepper

- 1/4 teaspoon lemon zest (rind), grated

- 1 1/2 pounds blue crab meat, flaked*

- 1/4 cup crab roe**

- 3 tablespoons dry sherry

- 1 tablespoon fresh parsley leaves, finely chopped

John Rutledge House Inn She Crab Soup:

- 5 tablespoons butter

- 1/2 cup celery, finely-chopped

- 2 cups crab meat***

- 3 1/2 cups milk

- 1/2 cup chicken stock

- 5 tablespoons all-purpose flour

- 2/3 teaspoon mace

- 1/4 teaspoon white pepper

- 1 cup heavy cream

- Salt to taste

- 1/4 cup Worcestershire Sauce

- 3 tablespoons sherry

- 2 eggs, hard-boiled and grated (optional)

- Paprika

Instructions

Charelston She Crab Soup Instructions:

In a large, heavy pot over low heat, melt butter; add flour and blend until smooth. Slowly add milk and half and half cream, stirring constantly with a whisk; cook until thickened.

Add onion, Worcestershire sauce, salt, white pepper, mace, cayenne pepper, and lemon zest. Bring just to a boil, stirring constantly. Reduce heat to low, add crabmeat and crab roe or crumbled hard-cooked egg yolks; simmer, uncovered, for 5 minutes (if the soup appears about to boil, remove the pan from the heat for a minute or so, then return).

Remove from heat and add sherry, stirring to mix. Let sit for 3 to 4 minutes before serving.

To serve, pour the soup into individual heated soup bowls, dividing the crabmeat and roe equally into each bowl.

Sprinkle with parsley and serve immediately.

Yields: 4 servings.

John Rutledge House Inn She Crab Soup Instructions:

Recipe courtesy of The John Rutledge House Inn.

In a large heavy pot over low heat, melt butter; add celery, mace, and white pepper. Cook until the celery is almost transparent.

In a small saucepan, while the celery is cooking, heat the milk and chicken stock until just hot, but not boiling.

When the celery mix is done cooking, stir in the flour to make a Roux-type mixture. Do not brown but heat enough to bubble for several minutes.

Slowly stir in the hot milk mixture and salt to the roux. Add the crab meat, cream, Worcestershire Sauce, and sherry. Let simmer for approximately 30 minutes or until thickened to appropriate consistency.

To serve, sprinkle with grated hard-boiled eggs and some paprika.

Yields: 8 servings.

Taverna Opa's Steamed King Crab Legs Recipe

Ingredients

- 1 tablespoon butter

- 2 tablespoons garlic, minced

- 3 cups (24-ounces) fish stock*

- 1 teaspoon salt

- 1 teaspoon black pepper, freshly-ground

- 2 1/2 pounds King Crab legs and claws, cooked and chilled, cracked and legs cut in half crosswise

- 1/2 cup 80-proof vodka, room temperature

- Clarified butter, melted

Instructions

Use a flambé pan, large skillet, or large chafing dish with rounded, deep sides and a long handle. Over medium, add the butter and let it melt. Add garlic and cook 1 1/2 minutes, until aromatic; do not let it burn. Add stock, salt, pepper, and crab legs. Cover and let simmer 6 minutes.

This may have to be done in batches if all the King Crab Legs do not all fit into the pan at one time. If done in batches, remove the heated legs from the pan and keep them warm until all are heated through. If done in batches, repeat until all are heated.

FlambeNote: If you are planning to flambé in front of your guests, light the dish at the table, but far away from guests and flammable objects. If you have a serving cart, now is the time to use it.

How To Flambe: When the last batch of crab legs are heated in the pan, remove cover, and reduce heat to medium high. Add the vodka around the sides of the pan and let the vodka warm. Ignite with a long match (such as fireplace matches or a long barbecue lighter). Never lean over the dish or pan as you light the fumes.

Let cook until flame disappears (at this point all alcohol has burned off).

Caution When You Flambe:

Please remember to use extreme caution here, you will be dealing with a liquid that is on fire.

Do not carry the dish while flaming, this is best done on a serving cart slightly away from your table.

Keep a large metal lid on hand, to cover the dish in case your flambé gets out of hand.

Once the flame subsides, serve crab legs with pan juices over them and a dish of melted clarified butter.

Makes 4 servings.

Hot Artichoke and Crab Appetizer Recipe

Ingredients

- 1/2 pound crab meat, cooked or 1 (6-ounce) can crab meat, drained

- 2/3 cup mayonnaise

- 1/2 cup artichoke hearts, marinated, drained, and chopped
- 1 teaspoon lemon juice, fresh-squeezed
- 1/2 cup Parmesan Cheese, freshly grated
- 1/4 cup onions, diced
- Baguette bread

Instructions

Preheat oven to 350 degrees F. If using fresh crab meat, carefully clean the crab meat of any shells or cartilage.

In an ungreased small 2-cup baking dish, combine crab meat, mayonnaise, artichoke hearts, lemon juice, parmesan cheese, and onion.

Bake, uncovered, 15 to 20 minutes or until thoroughly heated. Remove from oven and serve immediately with warm sliced baguette bread.

Makes 10 servings.

Gourmet Hot Crab Dip Recipe

Ingredients

- 1 pound crab meat, cooked*

- 1 (8-ounce) package cream cheese, softened

- 3 tablespoons sour cream

- 1 clove garlic, minced

- 1/2 cup celery, finely-chopped
- 1/2 cup green onions, finely-chopped
- 1 to 2 tablespoons lemon juice, fresh-squeezed
- 1 1/2 teaspoons horseradish, prepared
- 1 tablespoon Dijon mustard
- Few drops hot sauce, or to taste
- 1/4 cup Parmesan Cheese (Parmigiano-Reggiano), freshly-grated
- Coarse salt
- Baguette bread or crackers (of your choice)
- Green onion, chopped, for garnish

Instructions

Preheat oven to 350 degrees F.

In a medium-size bowl, combine cream cheese and sour cream until smooth and no lumps appears.

Stir into the cream cheese mixture the garlic, celery, green onion, lemon juice, horseradish, Dijon mustard, hot sauce, parmesan cheese, and Cayenne pepper.

Fold in the crab meat until well mixed. Add salt and adjust seasonings to taste.

Place the crab dip in an ungreased small 2-cup baking dish.

When ready to serve, bake for approximately 20 to 25 minutes or until top is bubbly and just starting to turn brown.

Garnish with sliced green onion, if desired. Serve with crackers or baguette bread slices.

Basil & lemon chickpeas with mackerel

Ingredients

- 3 tbsp olive oil , plus extra for drizzling

- 1 bunch spring onion , sliced

- 1 large garlic clove , crushed

- zest 1 lemon and squeeze of juice

- 2 x 400g can chickpeas , drained and rinsed

- 150ml vegetable stock

- 85g SunBlush tomato , halved

- 4 mackerel fillets, skin on

- 1 large bunch basil

Method

- STEP 1

Heat 2 tbsp oil in a large, shallow pan. Add the spring onions, garlic and lemon zest, then cook for 2 mins until the onions are tender but still very green. Add the chickpeas, then stir until well coated in the onion mixture. Lightly crush with a potato masher, then add the stock and tomatoes. Simmer for 3-4 mins or until the liquid is absorbed, then set aside to cool slightly.

- STEP 2

Meanwhile, heat the remaining oil in a large, non-stick frying pan over a medium heat. Season the mackerel fillets on both sides and fry for 3 mins each side, starting on the skin side. You'll probably need to cook these in two batches.

- STEP 3

Add the basil and a squeeze of lemon juice to the chickpeas, then season to taste. To serve, spoon the warm chickpeas onto serving plates, drizzle with a little extra olive oil and top with the mackerel fillets.

Easy Tomato Soup

EQUIPMENT

- Instant Pot (or stove top)
- Hand Blender (or regular blender)

INGREDIENTS

- 2 TBS cooking oil I like avocado & olive oil
- 1 small onion roughly diced
- 1-2 large garlic cloves minced
- 1 medium/large butternut squash peeled & roughly chopped
- 2 cups cranberries fresh or frozen
- 1 apple roughly chopped

- ½ TBS ginger powder
- ½ tsp cinnamon powder
- ¼ tsp mace
- ⅛ tsp cloves
- ½ tsp dried oregano
- ½ tsp dried basil
- ¼ tsp dried thyme
- ¼ tsp crushed dried rosemary
- ¾ tsp salt
- 5 cups bone broth

INSTRUCTIONS

1. Turn Instant Pot on "SAUTEE" and once hot add cooking oil.

2. Sautee onion until it begins to become translucent. Add garlic. Sautee for another couple of minutes. Turn "OFF"

3. Add the rest of the ingredients.

4. Press "SOUP" and time for 20 minutes.

5. You can quick or slow release – whatever is most convenient.

6. Use a hand blender (or a regular blender being careful since it's hot) to puree the soup. Enjoy!

7. If you don't have an Instant Pot, use a large stock pot and first sautee the onion and garlic and then add the rest of the ingredients (like above). Allow to simmer on the store until everything is well cooked through for easy blending. The Instant Pot concentrates flavors,

so you may need it to simmer a bit longer – perhaps an hour.

PASTA SALAD WITH BAKED TINGA SALMON

INGREDIENTS

- 75g gigli pasta (or any other pasta of choice)
- 1 small shallot, finely chopped
- 1 fat garlic clove, finely minced
- 80g edamame beans
- 50g cherry tomatoes, halved
- Large handful rocket
- 100g sliced sweet peppers
- 1/2 teaspoon dried thyme or 1 teaspoon mixed Italian herb

- 1 teaspoon olive oil

For the Salmon

- 2 medium salmon fillets, descaled
- 2 teaspoons Tinga paste

INSTRUCTIONS

1. Preheat the oven to 200ºC then line a baking tray with parchment paper. Season the salmon with a pinch of salt then coat evenly with the Tinga paste. Allow it to marinate in the fridge for 20-30 minutes then bake in the oven for 20 mins.

2. Start cooking the pasta according to the instructions. While the pasta cooks, heat the olive in a medium saucepan over medium heat.

Add the shallots, fry for 1 minute until fragrant. Add the garlic, fry for a half a minute then add the herbs, edamame, cherry tomatoes and sweet peppers. Fry for 3-4 minutes, stirring frequently.

3. Drain the pasta, reserving some of the cooking liquid. Tip the pasta into the veggie stir fry, mix throughly then season with salt or vegetable seasoning. Add a splash of the pasta liquid to loosen, if needed. Allow the pasta to cool for a few minutes before adding the rocket.

4. Serve the pasta salad with the salmon. Sprinkle with chilli flakes if desired.

Printed in the USA
CPSIA information can be obtained
at www.ICGtesting.com
LVHW012200021224
798164LV00039B/1162